MINDFUL
EATING

Tips for Healthier Eating Habits

Chew your food slowly,Focus on the food
on your plate and Use all of your senses
while eating.

by

Darlene Barton

Copyright © 2024 Darlene Barton

Table of contents

Introduction

Mindful eating is a practice that involves paying full attention to the experience of eating and drinking, both inside and outside the body. It involves being present in the moment, acknowledging all the senses—sight, smell, taste, touch, and even sound—while consuming food. Unlike mindless eating, where one may eat quickly and absentmindedly, mindful eating encourages a deeper connection with food, fostering a greater appreciation for the nourishment it provides.

What is Mindful Eating?

At its core, mindful eating is about bringing awareness to the eating process. It's about slowing down, savoring each bite, and truly tasting the flavors of the food. This practice encourages individuals to listen to their body's hunger and fullness cues, as well as to identify emotional triggers that may influence eating habits. Mindful eating isn't about restricting certain foods or following strict diets; rather, it's about developing a healthy relationship with food based on self-awareness and self-compassion.

Why Mindful Eating Matters

Mindful eating holds immense significance in today's fast-paced world where food consumption is often rushed and disconnected. Research has shown that practicing mindful eating can have numerous benefits for both physical and mental health. By paying attention to what and how much we eat, we can make healthier food choices, prevent overeating, and better manage weight. Moreover, mindful eating has been linked to improved digestion, reduced stress levels, and enhanced overall well-being.

In addition to its individual benefits, mindful eating also fosters a deeper appreciation for food and the process of eating. It encourages gratitude for the nourishment our meals provide and cultivates a sense of mindfulness in everyday life. Furthermore, mindful eating can contribute to a more sustainable food system by promoting mindful consumption and reducing food waste.

How This Book Can Help You

This book serves as a comprehensive guide to understanding and practicing mindful eating. Whether you're new to the concept or seeking to deepen your existing practice, the chapters within this book will provide you with valuable insights, practical techniques, and actionable strategies to incorporate mindful eating into your daily life.

Each chapter is designed to address different aspects of mindful eating, from the basic principles to practical techniques and overcoming challenges. By exploring topics such as setting the right environment for mindful eating, listening to your body's hunger and fullness cues, and overcoming common obstacles, you'll gain a holistic understanding of mindful eating and how it can benefit you.

Moreover, this book emphasizes the importance of self-compassion and flexibility in the journey toward mindful eating. It acknowledges that change takes time and encourages readers to approach the practice with kindness and patience. By offering a wealth of resources and support, this book aims to empower you to cultivate a healthier relationship with food and transform your eating habits for the better.

In essence, this book is not just about what to eat, but how to eat mindfully, with intention and awareness. It invites you to embark on a journey of self-discovery and self-care, where every meal becomes an opportunity to nourish your body, mind, and spirit. So, dive in, explore, and embrace the transformative power of mindful eating in your life.

Chapter 1

The Basics of Mindful Eating

Understanding the Principles of Mindful Eating

At its core, mindful eating is grounded in the principles of mindfulness—a practice that involves bringing one's attention to the present moment without judgment. When applied to eating, mindfulness transforms the act of consuming food into a mindful experience. Key principles of mindful eating include awareness, non-judgment, and acceptance. It's about being fully present while eating, paying attention to the sensations, thoughts, and emotions that arise without labeling them as good or bad.

One fundamental principle of mindful eating is listening to the body's hunger and fullness cues. This involves tuning in to the body's natural signals of hunger and satiety, rather than relying on external cues such as time of day or portion sizes. By eating when hungry and stopping when satisfied, individuals can develop a healthier relationship with food and prevent overeating.

Another principle of mindful eating is savoring the flavors and textures of food. This involves taking the time to truly taste and appreciate each bite, rather than mindlessly consuming food without awareness. By savoring the eating experience, individuals can derive greater pleasure and satisfaction from their meals, leading to a more fulfilling eating experience overall.

The Science Behind Mindful Eating

The practice of mindful eating is supported by a growing body of scientific research that highlights its numerous benefits for both physical and mental health. Studies have shown that mindful eating can lead to improved digestion, reduced stress levels, and better management of chronic conditions such as diabetes and heart disease. Additionally, research suggests that mindful eating may be effective in promoting weight loss and weight maintenance by encouraging healthier eating habits and reducing emotional eating.

One study published in the Journal of Obesity found that participants who underwent a mindfulness-based eating program experienced significant reductions in binge eating episodes and emotional eating behaviors compared to those who did not receive the intervention. Another study published in the American Journal of Clinical Nutrition found that mindfulness training was associated with reduced food cravings and increased awareness of hunger and fullness cues.

Neuroscientific research has also shed light on the mechanisms underlying mindful eating. Functional magnetic resonance imaging (fMRI) studies have shown that practicing mindfulness can lead to changes in brain activity associated with attention, emotion regulation, and self-awareness. These changes in brain function may help individuals become more attuned to their eating habits and make healthier choices.

Common Misconceptions About Eating Mindfully

Despite its growing popularity, mindful eating is often misunderstood or misrepresented. One common misconception is that mindful eating is synonymous with restrictive dieting or food rules. In reality, mindful eating is about fostering a positive and compassionate relationship with food, free from judgment or restriction. It encourages individuals to eat a wide variety of foods in moderation, while paying attention to their body's signals of hunger and fullness.

Another misconception is that mindful eating requires a significant time commitment or special training. While formal mindfulness practices such as meditation can enhance mindful eating skills, anyone can incorporate mindfulness into their eating habits with practice and intention. Simple techniques such as slowing down while eating, savoring each bite, and paying attention to the sensations of hunger and fullness can make a meaningful difference in one's relationship with food.

Overall, understanding the principles of mindful eating, appreciating the science behind it, and dispelling common misconceptions are essential steps in embracing this transformative practice. By cultivating awareness, acceptance, and compassion in our eating habits, we can nourish our bodies and minds more fully, leading to greater health and well-being.

Chapter 2

Preparing for Mindful Eating

Setting the Right Environment

Creating an environment conducive to mindful eating is essential for fostering a positive and enjoyable eating experience. This involves paying attention to factors such as lighting, noise level, and ambiance, which can influence our perception of food and our eating behaviors. For example, dimming harsh overhead lights and opting for softer, more natural lighting can create a relaxing atmosphere that encourages mindful eating. Similarly, minimizing distractions such as television, phones, and other electronic devices can help us focus our attention on the act of eating and fully appreciate the flavors and textures of our food. The social environment also plays a significant role in shaping our eating habits. Eating with others can enhance the enjoyment of meals and provide an opportunity for social connection, but it can also lead to mindless eating behaviours such as overeating or eating too quickly. By fostering a supportive and mindful eating environment, we can cultivate healthier eating habits and strengthen our relationships with food and with others.

Planning Your Meals Mindfully

Mindful meal planning involves more than just deciding what to eat; it's about considering how, when, and where we will eat our meals to optimize the mindful eating experience. This includes selecting a variety of nutritious foods that satisfy our taste preferences and dietary needs, as well as planning meals that are balanced in terms of macronutrients and micronutrients. By incorporating a diverse range of colors, flavors, and textures into our meals, we can make eating a more pleasurable and satisfying experience.

In addition to choosing nutritious foods, mindful meal planning also involves paying attention to portion sizes and serving methods. Instead of mindlessly piling food onto our plates, we can use visual cues such as the size of our hands or the proportions of different food groups to guide our portion sizes. Additionally, serving meals in smaller dishes or on smaller plates can help us avoid overeating by tricking our brains into perceiving larger portions as more satisfying.

Cultivating a Mindful Eating Mindset

Cultivating a mindful eating mindset is about adopting a curious, non-judgmental attitude toward food and eating. It involves letting go of rigid food rules and expectations and approaching each meal with openness and receptivity. This mindset encourages us to listen to our body's hunger and fullness cues, as well as to pay attention to how different foods make us feel physically, mentally, and emotionally.

One key aspect of cultivating a mindful eating mindset is practicing self-compassion. This involves treating ourselves with kindness and understanding, especially when we make choices that may not align with our health goals. Instead of berating ourselves for eating a "forbidden" food or overindulging at a meal, we can acknowledge our experiences without judgment and use them as opportunities for learning and growth.

Another important aspect of a mindful eating mindset is mindfulness itself—the practice of bringing our attention to the present moment with openness and curiosity. By cultivating mindfulness in our eating habits, we can become more attuned to the sensations, thoughts, and emotions that arise during meals, allowing us to make conscious choices that support our health and well-being. Preparing for mindful eating involves setting the right environment, planning meals mindfully, and cultivating a mindful eating mindset. By creating a supportive and nurturing environment for eating, selecting nutritious foods, and adopting a curious and non-judgmental attitude toward food and eating, we can enhance the mindful eating experience and reap the numerous benefits it offers for our health and well-being.

Chapter 3

Practical Techniques for Mindful Eating

Chewing Your Food Slowly

Chewing your food slowly is a foundational practice of mindful eating that can have profound effects on your overall eating experience and digestion. Many of us are accustomed to rushing through meals, often swallowing large chunks of food without fully chewing them. However, this habit can lead to a range of digestive issues, including bloating, gas, and indigestion. By chewing your food slowly and thoroughly, you give your digestive system the opportunity to break down food more efficiently, allowing for better nutrient absorption and smoother digestion.

When you chew your food slowly, you also give your brain more time to register signals of fullness, which can help prevent overeating and promote a greater sense of satisfaction from your meals. Additionally, chewing slowly allows you to fully experience the flavors and textures of your food, enhancing the sensory pleasure of eating. As you chew each bite mindfully, pay attention to the sensations in your mouth—the taste, texture, and temperature of the food—as well as the sound of your chewing. This heightened awareness can deepen your connection to the eating experience and foster a greater appreciation for the nourishment your food provides.

To incorporate the practice of chewing slowly into your meals, start by taking smaller bites and chewing each bite thoroughly before swallowing. Focus on the act of chewing, paying attention to the movement of your jaw and the sensations in your mouth. You may also find it helpful to put your utensils down between bites or to take a moment to pause and breathe before continuing to eat. With practice, chewing your food slowly will become a natural and intuitive part of your mindful eating routine, leading to improved digestion, enhanced satisfaction, and a greater sense of connection to your food.

Focusing on the Food on Your Plate

In today's fast-paced world, it's easy to eat mindlessly, with our attention divided between our meals and various distractions such as smartphones, computers, or television screens. However, when we focus our attention on the food on our plate, we can cultivate a deeper appreciation for the eating experience and make more conscious choices about what and how much we eat.

Focusing on the food on your plate involves engaging all of your senses—sight, smell, taste, touch, and even sound—to fully experience the flavors, textures, and aromas of your meal. Before taking your first bite, take a moment to pause and observe your food, noticing its colors, shapes, and arrangement on the plate. As you begin to eat, pay attention to the smells wafting from your dish, the sounds of your utensils against the plate, and the sensations of the food in your mouth.

By bringing mindfulness to the act of eating, you can savor each bite more fully and derive greater pleasure and satisfaction from your meals. Additionally, focusing on the food on your plate can help you become more attuned to your body's hunger and fullness cues, allowing you to eat more intuitively and in alignment with your body's needs.

To practice focusing on the food on your plate, try to minimize distractions during meals by turning off electronic devices, eating in a quiet environment, and giving yourself permission to fully immerse yourself in the eating experience. Take your time to chew each bite slowly and mindfully, paying attention to the sensations in your mouth and the flavors unfolding on your palate. With practice, you'll find that focusing on the food on your plate can enhance your enjoyment of meals and deepen your connection to the nourishment your food provides.

Engaging All Your Senses While Eating

Engaging all your senses while eating is a powerful way to bring mindfulness to the eating experience and deepen your connection to your food. Each of our senses plays a unique role in how we perceive and enjoy food, and by engaging all of them, we can enhance the sensory pleasure of eating and cultivate a greater appreciation for the nourishment our meals provide.

Start by taking a moment to observe your food with your eyes, noticing its colors, shapes, and textures. Allow yourself to appreciate the visual beauty of your meal before taking your first bite. As you begin to eat, pay attention to the aromas wafting from your dish, inhaling deeply to fully experience the scents. Notice how the smell of the food affects your anticipation and enjoyment of the meal.

Next, focus on the sensations of touch as you pick up your utensils and bring the food to your mouth. Notice the temperature and texture of the food against your lips and tongue, as well as the sensation of chewing and swallowing. Take your time to savor each bite, allowing yourself to fully experience the flavors unfolding on your palate.

Incorporating sound into the eating experience can also enhance mindfulness and sensory awareness. Pay attention to the sounds of your utensils against the plate, the crunch of vegetables, or the sizzle of food cooking.

These sounds can provide valuable feedback about the texture and freshness of your food, as well as add to the overall enjoyment of the meal.

Finally, don't forget to savor the taste of your food as you chew each bite slowly and mindfully. Notice the complex interplay of flavors on your palate—the sweetness of ripe fruit, the tanginess of fermented foods, the richness of savory dishes. Allow yourself to fully immerse in the sensory experience of eating, appreciating the nuances and subtleties of each flavor.

By engaging all your senses while eating, you can transform the act of eating into a mindful and pleasurable experience. This practice can help you become more attuned to your body's hunger and fullness cues, as well as deepen your appreciation for the nourishment and joy that food brings to your life.

Taking Time to Appreciate Your Food

Taking time to appreciate your food is a fundamental aspect of mindful eating that can profoundly impact your relationship with food and eating. In today's fast-paced world, it's easy to rush through meals or eat on the go, without taking the time to fully appreciate the flavors, textures, and nourishment that our food provides. However, by slowing down and intentionally savoring each bite, we can cultivate a deeper sense of gratitude and enjoyment for the meals we consume.

Appreciating your food involves more than just tasting it; it's about acknowledging the effort and care that went into preparing it, as well as recognizing the journey it took to reach your plate. Whether it's a home-cooked meal made with love, a fresh salad from the farmer's market, or a decadent dessert from your favorite bakery, each bite of food represents a unique opportunity to nourish and nurture your body and soul.

To practice taking time to appreciate your food, start by cultivating a sense of mindfulness and gratitude before each meal. Take a moment to pause and reflect on where your food came from, the people who grew, harvested, and prepared it, and the abundance of flavors and nutrients it offers. Allow yourself to fully immerse in the sensory experience of eating, savoring each bite with reverence and appreciation.

As you eat, pay attention to the sensations in your body and the emotions that arise, allowing yourself to fully experience the pleasure and nourishment of the meal. Take your time to chew each bite slowly and mindfully, noticing the flavors unfolding on your palate and the satisfaction that comes with each swallow. By taking time to appreciate your food, you can cultivate a deeper connection to the eating experience and foster a greater sense of fulfillment and contentment in your relationship with food and eating. Practical techniques for mindful eating such as chewing your food slowly, focusing on the food on your plate, engaging all your senses while eating, and taking time to appreciate your food are essential components of a mindful eating practice. These techniques help you slow down, become more present in the moment, and cultivate a deeper awareness of our eating habits and behaviors.

Chewing your food slowly allows you to fully break down food particles, aiding in digestion and allowing your body to absorb nutrients more effectively. By focusing on the food on your plate, you can heighten your sensory experience and become more attuned to your body's hunger and fullness cues. Engaging all your senses while eating enriches the eating experience, allowing you to fully savor the flavors, textures, and aromas of your food. Taking time to appreciate your food fosters a sense of gratitude and mindfulness, helping you develop a more positive relationship with food and eating.

Incorporating these practical techniques into your meals can have profound effects on your overall well-being. Not only can they improve digestion and nutrient absorption, but they can also help prevent overeating, reduce stress, and enhance the enjoyment of meals. By making mindful eating a regular part of your routine, you can cultivate a healthier and more balanced approach to food and eating, leading to greater satisfaction and vitality in your life.

Chapter 4

Listening to Your Body

Recognizing Hunger and Fullness Cues

One of the foundational principles of mindful eating is learning to recognize and respond to your body's hunger and fullness cues. In today's fast-paced world, it's easy to become disconnected from these natural signals, leading to overeating or undereating. However, by tuning in to your body's cues, you can develop a healthier and more intuitive approach to eating.

Hunger cues can manifest in a variety of ways, both physical and psychological. Physical cues may include stomach growling, low energy levels, or lightheadedness, while psychological cues may include thoughts or fantasies about food. Learning to identify and differentiate between physical and psychological hunger cues is key to developing a more mindful approach to eating.

Fullness cues, on the other hand, signal when your body has had enough food and is satisfied. These cues may include feelings of fullness or satisfaction, a decrease in appetite, or a loss of interest in food. By paying attention to these cues and stopping eating when you feel comfortably full, you can prevent overeating and promote greater balance and satisfaction in your eating habits.

To practice recognizing hunger and fullness cues, start by tuning in to your body's sensations before, during, and after meals. Before eating, take a moment to check in with yourself and assess your level of hunger. Are you experiencing physical sensations of hunger, such as a growling stomach or low energy levels? Or are you simply eating out of habit or boredom?

During meals, pay attention to how your hunger level changes as you eat. Notice when your hunger begins to diminish and when you start to feel satisfied or full. Take breaks between bites to check in with your body and assess your level of fullness. Aim to stop eating when you feel comfortably satisfied, rather than waiting until you feel overly full or stuffed.

By practicing mindful eating and listening to your body's hunger and fullness cues, you can develop a more balanced and harmonious relationship with food. Instead of relying on external cues or societal norms to dictate when and how much you eat, you can trust your body's innate wisdom to guide your eating decisions and support your overall health and well-being.

Understanding Emotional Eating

Emotional eating is a common phenomenon in which individuals use food to cope with or suppress negative emotions, such as stress, anxiety, sadness, or boredom. Unlike physical hunger, which is driven by the body's need for nourishment, emotional hunger is often triggered by psychological factors and can lead to mindless or excessive eating.

Emotional eating can take many forms, ranging from seeking comfort in high-calorie, "comfort" foods to mindlessly snacking as a way to distract from unpleasant emotions. While occasional emotional eating is a normal part of life, frequent or compulsive emotional eating can have negative consequences for both physical and emotional health, leading to weight gain, poor body image, and feelings of guilt or shame.

To understand and address emotional eating, it's important to recognize the underlying emotions and triggers that drive this behavior. This may involve becoming more aware of your emotional state and the patterns of behavior that accompany it. For example, do you tend to reach for food when you're feeling stressed or anxious? Are there certain situations or environments that trigger emotional eating for you?

Once you've identified your emotional triggers, you can begin to develop healthier coping strategies to address them. This may involve finding alternative ways to manage stress or anxiety, such as practicing relaxation techniques, engaging in physical activity, or seeking support from friends or loved ones. It may also involve learning to sit with and tolerate uncomfortable emotions without turning to food as a way to numb or distract yourself.

Strategies for Overcoming Emotional Eating

Overcoming emotional eating requires a multifaceted approach that addresses both the underlying emotions and the maladaptive eating behaviors associated with them. One strategy is to develop alternative coping mechanisms for dealing with difficult emotions. This may involve finding healthy ways to manage stress, such as practicing mindfulness meditation, journaling, or engaging in creative activities.

Another strategy is to cultivate greater self-awareness and mindfulness around eating habits. This may involve keeping a food diary to track when and why you eat, as well as identifying patterns or triggers that lead to emotional eating. By becoming more aware of your eating behaviors and the emotions that drive them, you can begin to make more conscious choices about how you respond to food cravings and urges.

In addition to addressing the emotional aspects of emotional eating, it's also important to cultivate a healthy relationship with food and body image. This may involve adopting a non-dieting approach to eating, in which you focus on nourishing your body with wholesome, satisfying foods rather than restricting or depriving yourself. It may also involve practicing self-compassion and acceptance, recognizing that occasional lapses in eating behavior are normal and forgivable.

Finally, seeking support from a therapist, counselor, or support group can be helpful for individuals struggling with emotional eating. Therapy can provide a safe space to explore underlying emotional issues and develop effective coping strategies for managing them. Additionally, connecting with others who share similar experiences can provide validation, encouragement, and accountability in your journey toward overcoming emotional eating. Listening to your body involves recognizing hunger and fullness cues, understanding emotional eating, and developing strategies for overcoming it. By tuning in to your body's signals, becoming more aware of emotional triggers, and cultivating healthier coping mechanisms, you can develop a more balanced and mindful approach to eating that supports your overall health and well-being.

Chapter 5

Overcoming Challenges

Dealing with Distractions While Eating

In today's fast-paced world, it's all too easy to succumb to distractions while eating. Whether it's scrolling through your phone, watching TV, or working at your desk, distractions can prevent you from fully experiencing and enjoying your meals. Not only can this lead to mindless eating and overeating, but it can also detract from the pleasure and satisfaction of the eating experience.

To overcome distractions while eating, it's important to cultivate mindfulness and presence at the table. This may involve creating a designated eating space free from electronic devices and other distractions, where you can focus solely on the act of eating and the sensory experience of your meal. Set aside time for meals without any other activities or tasks competing for your attention, and practice eating in silence or with soft background music to minimize distractions.

Another strategy for dealing with distractions while eating is to practice mindful eating techniques, such as chewing slowly and savoring each bite. By bringing your attention to the sensations of eating—the taste, texture, and aroma of your food—you can anchor yourself in the present moment and reduce the tendency to become distracted by external stimuli. Additionally, taking breaks between bites to check in with yourself and assess your level of hunger and fullness can help prevent mindless eating and promote greater awareness of your body's needs.

Overcoming Cravings and Temptations

Cravings and temptations are a common challenge when it comes to mindful eating, especially in a culture saturated with highly palatable, processed foods. Whether it's a craving for something sweet, salty, or savory, resisting the urge to indulge can be difficult, particularly when faced with triggers such as stress, boredom, or social situations. However, with practice and perseverance, it is possible to overcome cravings and make more conscious choices about what and how much you eat.

One strategy for overcoming cravings is to identify the underlying cause and address it directly. For example, if you find yourself craving sweets when you're feeling stressed, finding alternative ways to manage stress, such as deep breathing exercises or taking a walk, can help reduce the intensity of the craving. Similarly, if you tend to crave certain foods when you're bored or lonely, finding ways to engage in meaningful activities or connect with others can help distract you from the urge to eat.

Another strategy for overcoming cravings is to practice mindful eating techniques, such as bringing awareness to the sensations of hunger and fullness and savoring each bite of food. By slowing down and paying attention to the flavors and textures of your food, you can satisfy your cravings more mindfully and with smaller portions, reducing the likelihood of overindulging. Additionally, incorporating more whole, nutrient-dense foods into your diet can help reduce cravings for processed, unhealthy foods over time.

Handling Social Situations and Peer Pressure

Social situations and peer pressure can present significant challenges when it comes to mindful eating. Whether it's navigating office gatherings, family dinners, or social outings with friends, the pressure to conform to social norms and expectations around food can make it difficult to stay true to your mindful eating goals. However, with some awareness and planning, it is possible to navigate these situations in a way that aligns with your values and priorities.

One strategy for handling social situations and peer pressure is to communicate your intentions and boundaries with others. Letting friends, family members, and coworkers know that you're committed to mindful eating and may make different food choices than they do can help set clear expectations and reduce the pressure to conform. Additionally, offering to bring a dish or snack to social gatherings that aligns with your dietary preferences can ensure that you have healthy options available to you.

Another strategy is to practice assertiveness and self-advocacy in social situations. If you're faced with peer pressure to eat or drink something that doesn't align with your mindful eating goals, politely but firmly decline and offer an alternative explanation or suggestion. For example, you might say something like, "Thank you, but I'm trying to be more mindful of my eating habits lately, so I'll pass on the dessert. How about we go for a walk instead?"

Furthermore, finding support from like-minded individuals or joining a community of people who share similar values and goals around food and eating can provide encouragement, accountability, and validation in your journey toward mindful eating. Whether it's through online forums, social media groups, or local meetups, connecting with others who understand and support your mindful eating journey can help you stay motivated and resilient in the face of social pressures and challenges. Overcoming challenges such as dealing with distractions while eating, managing cravings and temptations, and handling social situations and peer pressure requires a combination of mindfulness, self-awareness, and assertiveness. By practicing mindful eating techniques, identifying and addressing underlying triggers, and seeking support from others, you can navigate these challenges with greater ease and confidence, ultimately cultivating a healthier and more balanced relationship with food and eating.

Chapter 6

Nourishing Your Body and Mind

Choosing Nutrient-Dense Foods

Nourishing your body with nutrient-dense foods is essential for supporting overall health and well-being. Nutrient-dense foods are those that provide a high concentration of essential nutrients—such as vitamins, minerals, protein, and fiber—relative to their calorie content. By choosing a variety of nutrient-dense foods, you can ensure that your body receives the essential nutrients it needs to function optimally and thrive.

When it comes to selecting nutrient-dense foods, focus on incorporating a colorful array of fruits and vegetables into your diet. These plant-based foods are rich in vitamins, minerals, antioxidants, and phytochemicals that support immune function, reduce inflammation, and protect against chronic diseases such as heart disease, diabetes, and cancer. Aim to fill half your plate with fruits and vegetables at each meal, choosing a variety of colors and types to maximize nutrient intake.

In addition to fruits and vegetables, prioritize whole grains, lean proteins, and healthy fats in your diet. Whole grains such as quinoa, brown rice, and oats are rich in fiber, vitamins, and minerals, while lean proteins such as poultry, fish, beans, and tofu provide essential amino acids for muscle growth and repair. Healthy fats found in avocados, nuts, seeds, and olive oil are important for brain health, hormone production, and absorption of fat-soluble vitamins.

When choosing packaged or processed foods, opt for options that are minimally processed and contain simple, recognizable ingredients. Avoid foods that are high in added sugars, sodium, and unhealthy fats, as these can contribute to inflammation, weight gain, and chronic disease risk. Instead, look for products with short ingredient lists and minimal additives or preservatives.

Mindful Eating for Weight Management

Mindful eating can be a powerful tool for weight management, helping you make more conscious choices about what and how much you eat. Unlike restrictive diets or calorie counting, mindful eating focuses on cultivating awareness, listening to your body's hunger and fullness cues, and eating with intention and attention. By practicing mindful eating, you can develop a healthier relationship with food and eating, leading to more sustainable weight loss and maintenance.

One key aspect of mindful eating for weight management is paying attention to portion sizes and serving sizes. Instead of relying on external cues such as plate size or portion recommendations, tune in to your body's hunger and fullness cues to determine how much food you need to feel satisfied. Eat slowly and mindfully, taking breaks between bites to check in with your body and assess your level of fullness.

Another important aspect of mindful eating for weight management is becoming more attuned to the reasons behind your eating habits. Are you eating out of physical hunger, emotional hunger, or simply out of habit or boredom? By identifying and addressing the underlying emotions and triggers that drive your eating behaviors, you can develop healthier coping strategies and make more conscious choices about when and what you eat.

In addition to paying attention to what you eat, also consider how you eat. Mindful eating encourages you to eat without distractions, savoring each bite and fully experiencing the flavors and textures of your food. By bringing mindfulness to the eating experience, you can enhance satisfaction and enjoyment, leading to a greater sense of fulfillment and contentment with your meals.

Incorporating Mindfulness Beyond Meal Times

While mindful eating primarily focuses on the act of eating, mindfulness can be incorporated into other aspects of daily life as well. By bringing mindfulness to activities such as cooking, grocery shopping, and food preparation, you can deepen your connection to the food you eat and enhance the overall eating experience.

When cooking or preparing meals, practice mindfulness by focusing on the sensations, smells, and sounds of the cooking process. Take a moment to appreciate the colors and textures of the ingredients, and engage your senses as you chop, sauté, and season your dishes. Cooking mindfully can not only enhance the flavor and enjoyment of your meals but also foster a greater sense of creativity and satisfaction in the kitchen.

Similarly, practice mindfulness when grocery shopping by paying attention to the sights, smells, and sounds of the supermarket. Take your time to explore different aisles and sections of the store, and choose fresh, whole foods that nourish your body and support your health goals. Avoid shopping when hungry or stressed, as this can lead to impulsive food choices and overeating.

Beyond meal times, incorporate mindfulness into other aspects of your daily routine, such as physical activity, relaxation, and self-care practices. Whether it's practicing yoga, going for a walk in nature, or simply taking a few moments to pause and breathe deeply, mindfulness can help you become more present and centered in the moment, reducing stress and enhancing overall well-being. Nourishing your body and mind involves choosing nutrient-dense foods, practicing mindful eating for weight management, and incorporating mindfulness beyond meal times. By focusing on nourishing your body with wholesome, nutrient-rich foods, listening to your body's hunger and fullness cues, and bringing mindfulness to all aspects of the eating experience, you can cultivate a healthier and more balanced relationship with food and eating, leading to greater health and vitality in body and mind.

Chapter 7

Cultivating Lasting Habits

Making Mindful Eating a Sustainable Practice

Making mindful eating a sustainable practice involves integrating it into your daily life in a way that feels manageable and enjoyable. Rather than viewing mindful eating as a short-term diet or trend, approach it as a long-term lifestyle change that supports your overall health and well-being. To make mindful eating sustainable, it's important to start small and gradually build upon your successes over time.

Begin by incorporating mindful eating into one meal or snack each day, focusing on bringing awareness to the eating experience and savoring each bite. As you become more comfortable with mindful eating, gradually expand the practice to other meals and snacks throughout the day. Remember that progress is not always linear, and it's okay to have setbacks or challenges along the way. The key is to approach each meal with curiosity and openness, and to be gentle with yourself as you navigate the process.

Another strategy for making mindful eating sustainable is to set realistic goals and expectations. Rather than aiming for perfection or strict adherence to rigid rules, focus on making small, incremental changes that are sustainable over the long term. For example, instead of completely eliminating your favorite indulgence foods, aim to enjoy them mindfully and in moderation, savoring each bite and being present in the eating experience.

In addition to setting realistic goals, it's important to cultivate a positive mindset and self-talk around mindful eating. Rather than viewing mindful eating as a chore or obligation, approach it with a sense of curiosity, openness, and self-compassion. Celebrate your successes and acknowledge your efforts, even if progress feels slow or incremental. Remember that every small step you take toward mindful eating is a step in the right direction toward greater health and well-being.

Building a Supportive Environment

Building a supportive environment is essential for cultivating lasting habits and sustaining mindful eating practices. Surrounding yourself with supportive friends, family members, and communities can provide encouragement, accountability, and motivation as you navigate the challenges and obstacles of mindful eating.

Additionally, creating a physical environment that supports mindful eating can help reinforce your commitment to the practice and make it easier to stay on track.

One way to build a supportive environment for mindful eating is to involve friends and family members in the process. Share your goals and intentions with loved ones, and enlist their support in your mindful eating journey. Encourage family meals and cooking together, and involve others in meal planning and preparation. By fostering a supportive and collaborative atmosphere around food and eating, you can create a sense of shared responsibility and accountability for making healthy choices.

In addition to involving others in your mindful eating journey, create a physical environment that supports your goals and priorities. Stock your kitchen with healthy, nutrient-dense foods and minimize the presence of highly processed, unhealthy options. Arrange your kitchen and dining space in a way that promotes mindfulness and enjoyment during meals, such as setting a beautiful table, using smaller plates and utensils, and minimizing distractions such as television or electronic devices.

Another way to build a supportive environment for mindful eating is to seek out resources and support from like-minded individuals and communities. Whether it's joining a mindful eating group, participating in online forums or social media groups, or attending workshops or classes, connecting with others who share similar values and goals around food and eating can provide encouragement, inspiration, and validation in your mindful eating journey.

Monitoring Progress and Adjusting Strategies

Monitoring progress and adjusting strategies is an essential part of cultivating lasting habits and sustaining mindful eating practices. Regularly assessing your progress, identifying areas for improvement, and making adjustments as needed can help you stay on track and continue moving toward your goals over time. Rather than viewing setbacks or challenges as failures, see them as opportunities for learning and growth, and use them to refine your approach and strengthen your commitment to mindful eating.

One strategy for monitoring progress is to keep a food diary or journal to track your eating habits, thoughts, and emotions around food, and experiences with mindful eating. Note any patterns or trends you observe, such as times of day when you tend to eat mindlessly or triggers that lead to emotional eating. Use this information to identify areas for improvement and develop strategies for addressing them, such as finding alternative coping mechanisms for stress or boredom, or planning ahead for challenging situations.

In addition to keeping a food diary, regularly check in with yourself and assess your level of mindfulness and presence during meals. Notice any moments of mindlessness or distraction, and reflect on what may have contributed to them. Use this awareness to make adjustments to your eating environment, routines, or habits as needed, and to recommit to the practice of mindful eating with renewed focus and intention.

Finally, be open to experimenting with different mindful eating techniques and strategies to find what works best for you. Not every approach will resonate with every person, so it's important to be flexible and adaptable in your approach. Be willing to try new things, and be patient with yourself as you navigate the process of cultivating lasting habits and sustaining mindful eating practices. Remember that progress takes time, and that every small step you take toward mindful eating is a step in the right direction toward greater health and well-being.

Conclusion

As you reach the conclusion of your mindful eating journey, take a moment to reflect on how far you've come and the progress you've made toward cultivating a healthier and more balanced relationship with food and eating. Throughout this journey, you've explored the principles and practices of mindful eating, learned to recognize and respond to your body's hunger and fullness cues, and navigated the challenges and obstacles that arise along the way. Now, as you prepare to move forward with confidence and awareness, it's important to take stock of your experiences and insights, and to commit to continuing your mindful eating journey with intention and purpose.

Reflecting on Your Mindful Eating Journey

Reflecting on your mindful eating journey allows you to acknowledge and celebrate your accomplishments, as well as to identify areas for further growth and development. Take some time to consider the ways in which mindful eating has impacted your life, both physically and emotionally. Notice any changes in your eating habits, attitudes toward food, or overall sense of well-being since beginning this journey. Perhaps you've become more attuned to your body's hunger and fullness cues, or discovered new ways to cope with stress and emotional eating. Whatever insights you've gained, honor and appreciate them as valuable lessons learned along the way.

Reflecting on your mindful eating journey also involves recognizing the challenges and obstacles you've encountered, and the strategies you've used to overcome them. Recall the times when you felt tempted to revert to old habits or patterns of behavior, and the moments when you chose to stay committed to your mindful eating goals. Consider the support systems and resources that have helped you along the way, whether it's the encouragement of friends and family, the guidance of a mentor or teacher, or the wisdom of books and articles on mindful eating. Acknowledge and express gratitude for the people and resources that have supported you on your journey, and use their encouragement and wisdom as sources of strength and inspiration moving forward.

In addition to reflecting on your past experiences, take some time to envision the future you want to create for yourself in relation to food and eating. What are your hopes, dreams, and aspirations for your mindful eating practice? How do you envision your relationship with food and eating evolving and deepening over time? Set intentions and goals for yourself that are aligned with your values and priorities, and commit to taking concrete actions to manifest them in your life. Whether it's incorporating new mindful eating techniques and practices into your daily routine, or seeking out additional support and resources to further your journey, trust in your ability to create the life you desire and deserve.

Moving Forward with Confidence and Awareness

As you prepare to move forward with confidence and awareness on your mindful eating journey, remember that you are the author of your own story, and that you have the power to shape your relationship with food and eating in a way that honors your body, mind, and spirit. Embrace the lessons and insights you've gained along the way, and carry them with you as guiding lights on your path forward. Trust in your intuition and inner wisdom to lead you toward choices and decisions that support your health and well-being, and cultivate a sense of curiosity, openness, and self-compassion as you navigate the ups and downs of life.

Moving forward with confidence and awareness also involves cultivating a sense of resilience and adaptability in the face of challenges and obstacles. Recognize that setbacks and setbacks are a natural part of any journey, and that they can serve as opportunities for growth and learning. Instead of viewing them as failures or shortcomings, reframe them as valuable lessons and opportunities for self-discovery and personal growth. Approach each new challenge with a sense of curiosity and openness, and trust in your ability to overcome them with grace and resilience.

In addition to resilience and adaptability, moving forward with confidence and awareness requires a commitment to self-care and self-compassion. Prioritize your physical, emotional, and spiritual well-being, and take time each day to nourish and nurture yourself in body, mind, and spirit. Whether it's through meditation, exercise, journaling, or spending time in nature, find practices that replenish and rejuvenate you, and make them a regular part of your self-care routine. Cultivate a sense of self-compassion and acceptance toward yourself, and treat yourself with kindness, patience, and understanding as you navigate the ups and downs of life.

In summary, the conclusion of your mindful eating journey is an opportunity to reflect on your experiences, celebrate your accomplishments, and envision the future you want to create for yourself in relation to food and eating. By reflecting on your past experiences, setting intentions and goals for the future, and moving forward with confidence and awareness, you can continue to cultivate a healthier and more balanced relationship with food and eating, and create a life that nourishes and supports you in body, mind, and spirit. Trust in yourself and the wisdom of your own inner guidance, and know that you have everything you need to thrive on your mindful eating journey.